WOMEN'S GUIDE TO STRENGTH TRAINING

PLUS

A 12 WEEKS WORKOUT

PLAN

Copyright © 2023

Sam's Fitness Club
doctorsam191@yahoo.com

CONTENT

Introduction

1). What is Strength Training?
I) benefits of strength training

2). 20 motivational quotes for strength training

3). 12 weeks workout plan

Introduction

In a world where strength knows no gender, where empowerment takes center stage, and where resilience is celebrated, the **"Women's Guide To Strength Training"** emerges as a beacon of transformation and empowerment. Welcome to a journey that will redefine the way you perceive fitness, redefine your body, and redefine your life.

In these pages, we will embark on a voyage to unveil the profound benefits of strength training specifically tailored for women. Whether you're a beginner, an athlete, or someone looking to rekindle their passion for fitness, this guide will be your trusted companion.

1. What is Strength Training?

Strength training, also known as resistance training or weight training, is a type of physical exercise that focuses on improving muscular strength, endurance, and overall fitness. It involves performing exercises that use resistance, such as weights, resistance bands, or body weight, to challenge and stimulate the muscles.

The main goal of strength training is to increase muscle mass, improve muscular strength, and enhance functional fitness. This type of training involves progressively increasing the resistance or weight used in exercises, which helps the muscles adapt and grow stronger over time. Strength training can target specific muscle groups or the entire body, and it can be tailored to various fitness levels and goals.

I). Benefit of Strength Training

1. Increases Muscle Strength: By progressively challenging the muscles, strength training leads to increased muscle strength and power.

2. Enhances Bone Health: Strength training helps improve bone density and reduce the risk of osteoporosis.

3. Improves Metabolism: Building muscle through strength training can boost metabolism, aiding in weight management and fat loss.

4. Better Joint Health: Strengthening the muscles around joints can provide better support and reduce the risk of injury.

5. Enhances Functional Fitness: Stronger muscles improve everyday activities and overall physical performance.

6. Increases Confidence: Achieving strength and fitness goals can boost self-esteem and confidence.

7. Injury Prevention: Strength training can help correct imbalances and weaknesses that might lead to injuries.

8. Long-Term Health: Regular strength training is associated with a reduced risk of chronic conditions like heart disease, diabetes, and more.

2). 20 motivational quotes To Fuel Your Strength Training Journey

1. "The only bad workout is the one that didn't happen."

2. "Strength doesn't come from what you can do; it comes from overcoming the things you once thought you couldn't."

3. "Pain is temporary, pride is forever."

4. "Don't wish for it, work for it."

5. "Success is the sum of small efforts repeated day in and day out."

6. "You don't have to be great to start, but you have to start to be great."

7. "The body achieves what the mind believes."

8. "Train insane or remain the same."

9. "Champions aren't made in the gyms. Champions are made from something they have deep inside them: a desire, a dream, a vision."

10. "Sweat is fat crying."

11. "It never gets easier, you just get stronger."

12. "The pain you feel today will be the strength you feel tomorrow."

13. "Your body can stand almost anything. It's your mind that you have to convince."

14. "Strength training is about progress, not perfection."

15. "The harder you work for something, the greater you'll feel when you achieve it."

16. "Limits exist only in the mind."

17. "Make your effort count, because each drop of sweat brings you closer to your goals."

18. "Every day is another chance to get stronger, to eat better, to live healthier, and to be the best version of you."

19. "Doubt kills more dreams than failure ever will."

20. "Remember why you started."

Stay motivated and keep pushing yourself towards your strength training goals!

NB:

Strength training exercises can range from lifting weights and using resistance machines to bodyweight exercises like push-ups, squats, and planks. It's important to follow proper form and technique to prevent injury and achieve the best results. Whether you're a beginner or experienced athlete, incorporating strength training into your fitness routine can contribute to a healthier and stronger body.

Every exercise in the workout
plan
will be explained to it's detail.
Thereby letting you
know what muscle group
it targets and how to perform
them with perfect form and
technique.

3). 12 WEEKS WORKOUT PLAN/ROUTINE

Here's a 12-week strength training workout plan for women. This plan is designed to help you progressively build strength and muscle over the course of 12 weeks. Remember to adjust the weights and repetitions according to your fitness level, and always prioritize proper form and technique.

Weeks 1-4: Foundation and Technique

Day 1: Full Body

- Squats: 3 sets of 10 reps
- Push-ups (or knee push-ups): 3 sets of 8 reps
- Bent-over Dumbbell Rows: 3 sets of 10 reps
- Plank: 3 sets of 20-30 seconds

Day 2: Rest or Light Cardio

1). SQUATS

primarily target the muscles in the lower body, particularly the following muscle groups:

1. **Quadriceps:** The quadriceps, located on the front of the thighs, are the primary muscles engaged during squats. They are responsible for extending the knee joint as you stand up from a squatting position.

2. **Hamstrings:** The hamstrings, situated on the back of the thighs, act as stabilizers during squats and assist in controlling the descent phase of the movement.

3. **Glutes:** The gluteal muscles, including the gluteus maximus, medius, and minimus, play a significant role in hip extension during the upward phase of the squat. This is especially true when you stand up from the squatting position.

4. **Calves:** The calf muscles help with stabilization during the movement, and they assist in pushing off the ground as you rise from the squat.

5. **Core:** Your core muscles, the abdominals and lower back muscles, are engaged to stabilize your torso throughout the squatting motion.

6. **Adductors and Abductors:** The adductor muscles on the inside of the thighs and the abductor muscles on the outside of the hips help stabilize the legs during the squatting movement.

Squats are a compound exercise, meaning they involve multiple muscle groups working together. They are an excellent way to strengthen and tone the lower body, enhance functional fitness, and improve overall lower body strength and stability.

2). PUSH –UPS

are a compound bodyweight exercise that primarily work the muscles of the upper body. Here are the main muscle groups targeted during pushups:

1. **Chest (Pectoralis Major):** Push-ups heavily engage the chest muscles, which are responsible for the horizontal movement of your arms. They help push your body away from the ground.

2. **Shoulders (Deltoids):** The anterior deltoid muscles at the front of your shoulders are actively involved in the pushing motion of push-ups.

3. **Triceps:** The back of your upper arms, known as the triceps, are engaged as you extend your elbows to push your body up.

4. **Core (Abdominals and Lower Back):** Your core muscles are essential for maintaining a straight and stable body position during push-ups. They help prevent excessive arching or sagging of the lower back.

5. **Serratus Anterior:** This muscle runs along the sides of your ribcage and helps stabilize the shoulder blades during the movement.

6. **Scapular Stabilizers (Rhomboids and Trapezius):** The muscles between your shoulder blades and upper back play a role in stabilizing the shoulder girdle as you perform push-ups.

While push-ups primarily target these muscle groups, they also engage other stabilizing muscles throughout the body, such as the lower body muscles, to help maintain a proper plank position during the movement. Push-ups are versatile and can be modified to suit different fitness levels, making them an effective bodyweight exercise for building upper body strength and stability.

3). BENT OVER DUMBBELL ROWS

Bent over dumbbell rows primarily target the muscles in your upper back, including the latissimus dorsi, rhomboids, and trapezius muscles. They also engage the biceps and lower back muscles to some extent.

4). PLANKS

Planks primarily target the core muscles, including the rectus abdominis (front of the abdomen), transverse abdominis (deep core muscles), obliques (side of the abdomen), and the muscles that support the lower back. They also engage muscles in the shoulders, chest, and legs to help maintain proper alignment.

5). CARDIO

Cardiovascular exercise, often referred to as "cardio," has several positive effects on the body. It helps strengthen the heart and improve its efficiency in pumping blood. Cardio also enhances lung function, increasing oxygen delivery to tissues and improving overall respiratory health. It aids in burning calories and fat, contributing to weight management. Regular cardio can improve circulation, reduce the risk of chronic diseases like heart disease and diabetes, boost mood through the release of endorphins, and increase stamina and endurance.

Day 3: Lower Body

- Deadlifts (or Romanian Deadlifts): 3 sets of 8 reps
- Lunges (each leg): 3 sets of 10 reps
- Glute Bridges: 3 sets of 12 reps

Day 4: Rest or Light Cardio

1). ROMANIAN DEADLIFT

A Romanian deadlift (RDL) is a strength training exercise that targets the muscles in the posterior chain, primarily the hamstrings, glutes, and lower back. Here's how to perform it:

1. Stand with your feet hip-width apart, holding a barbell or dumbbells in front of your thighs, palms facing your body.

2. Keep your knees slightly bent and maintain a straight posture with your chest up and shoulders back.

3. While keeping a slight bend in your knees, hinge at your hips and lower the weights by pushing your hips back.

4. Lower the weights down the front of your legs while maintaining a straight back, allowing the weights to move as far down your legs as your flexibility allows.

5. Feel a stretch in your hamstrings, but avoid rounding your back.

6. Once you feel a comfortable stretch or your back begins to round, reverse the movement by pushing your hips forward and returning to the starting position.

Remember to keep your core engaged throughout the movement to protect your lower back. Proper form is crucial to prevent injury and effectively target the intended muscle groups.

2). LUNGES

Lunges are a common strength training exercise that targets the lower body muscles, including the quadriceps, hamstrings, glutes, and calves. Here's how to perform a basic lunge:

1. Stand tall with your feet hip-width apart.

2. Take a step forward with one leg, lowering your body until both knees are bent at roughly 90-degree angles. The back knee should hover just above the ground.

3. Keep your upper body upright, with your chest lifted and shoulders relaxed.

4. Push through the heel of your front foot to return to the starting position.

5. Repeat on the other leg.

Lunges can be performed in various directions (forward, reverse, or to the side) and can be modified by adding weights or other variations to increase the intensity. They help improve lower body strength, stability, and balance while engaging multiple muscle groups.

3). GLUTES BRIDGES

Glute bridges are a lower body exercise that primarily targets the gluteal muscles (also known as the "glutes"). Here's how to perform a glute bridge:

1. Lie on your back with your knees bent and feet flat on the floor, hip-width apart.

2. Keep your arms by your sides, palms facing down.

3. Engage your core muscles
and squeeze your glutes.

4. Press through your heels
and lift your hips off the
ground, creating a straight
line from your shoulders to
your knees.

5. Hold the position at the top
for a second, focusing on
squeezing your glutes.

6. Lower your hips back down to the ground with control.

Glute bridges help strengthen the glutes, hamstrings, and lower back muscles, and they can also contribute to better hip mobility and posture. They can be done as part of a workout routine or as a warm-up exercise.

Day 5: Upper Body

- Bench Press (or Dumbbell Press): 3 sets of 8 reps
- Lat Pulldowns (or Assisted Pull-ups): 3 sets of 10 reps
- Dumbbell Shoulder Press: 3 sets of 10 reps

Day 6: Rest or Light Cardio

Day 7: Rest

1). BENCH PRESS

A bench press is a classic strength training exercise that targets the muscles of the chest, shoulders, and triceps. It is typically performed using a bench and a barbell or dumbbells. Here's how to do a bench press with a barbell:

1. Lie flat on a bench with your feet planted on the floor and your eyes directly under the barbell.

2. Grip the barbell slightly wider than shoulder-width apart, with your palms facing away from your body.

3. Unrack the barbell and lower it slowly towards your chest, keeping your elbows at around a 45-degree angle.

4. Touch your chest lightly with the barbell, then push it back up to the starting position, extending your arms fully.

5. Repeat for the desired number of repetitions.

Bench presses help develop upper body strength, particularly in the chest, shoulders, and triceps. They can be varied by using different equipment or angles, and they are a fundamental exercise in many weightlifting routines.

2. LATS PULLDOWN

Lat pulldowns are a strength training exercise that targets the latissimus dorsi muscles, commonly known as the "lats." The exercise is performed using a lat pulldown machine or a cable machine with a high pulley attachment. Here's how to do lat pulldowns:

1. Sit down on the lat pulldown machine and secure your legs under the thigh pads.

2. Grip the bar overhead, with your hands slightly wider than shoulder-width apart and palms facing forward (overhand grip).

3. Sit down with your back straight and a slight lean back in your torso.

4. Pull the bar down towards your upper chest, while squeezing your shoulder blades together.

5. Pause briefly when the bar is close to your chest, then slowly release it back up to the starting position, fully extending your arms.

6. Maintain a controlled and smooth motion throughout the exercise.

Lat pulldowns primarily target the lats, which are large muscles on the sides of your back. They also engage other muscles in the upper back, shoulders, and arms, making it a beneficial exercise for overall upper body strength and development.

3. DUMBBELL SHOULDER PRESS

A dumbbell shoulder press, also known as a dumbbell overhead press, is a strength training exercise that targets the shoulder muscles, specifically the deltoids. Here's how to perform a dumbbell shoulder press:

1. Sit on a bench with back support or stand with your feet shoulder-width apart.

2. Hold a dumbbell in each hand at shoulder height, with your palms facing forward and your elbows bent.

3. Press the dumbbells overhead by extending your arms fully, while keeping your core engaged and maintaining a neutral spine.

4. Lower the dumbbells back down to shoulder height in a controlled manner.

Dumbbell shoulder presses help develop shoulder strength, stability, and muscle definition. They work the anterior (front), lateral (side), and posterior (rear) deltoid muscles, as well as the trapezius and triceps to some extent. It's important to use proper form and start with an appropriate weight to prevent strain or injury.

Weeks 5-8: Increasing Intensity

Increase the weights slightly and aim to perform an additional set for each exercise.

Weeks 9-12: Advanced Strength

Day 1: Full Body

- Squats: 4 sets of 8 reps
- Push-ups (or knee push-ups): 4 sets of 6 reps
- Bent-over Dumbbell Rows: 4 sets of 8 reps
- Plank: 4 sets of 30-40 seconds

Day 2: Rest or Light Cardio

Day 3: Lower Body

- Deadlifts (or Romanian Deadlifts): 4 sets of 6 reps
- Lunges (each leg): 4 sets of 8 reps
- Glute Bridges: 4 sets of 10 reps

Day 4: Rest or Light Cardio

Day 5: Upper Body

- Bench Press (or Dumbbell Press): 4 sets of 6 reps
- Lat Pulldowns (or Assisted Pull-ups): 4 sets of 8 reps
- Dumbbell Shoulder Press: 4 sets of 8 reps

Day 6: Rest or Light Cardio

Day 7: Rest

NB:
Throughout the entire 12-week period, focus on progressive overload by gradually increasing the weights as you become stronger. Always warm up before each workout, cool down afterward, and prioritize recovery with proper nutrition and adequate sleep. Before starting any new workout plan, consult a fitness professional or healthcare provider, especially if you have any pre-existing health conditions or concerns.

www.ingramcontent.com/pod-product-compliance
Lightning Source LLC
Chambersburg PA
CBHW070728260726
48660CB00007B/2771